# The Magic of Coffee

### Knowing More about Coffee

I0435674

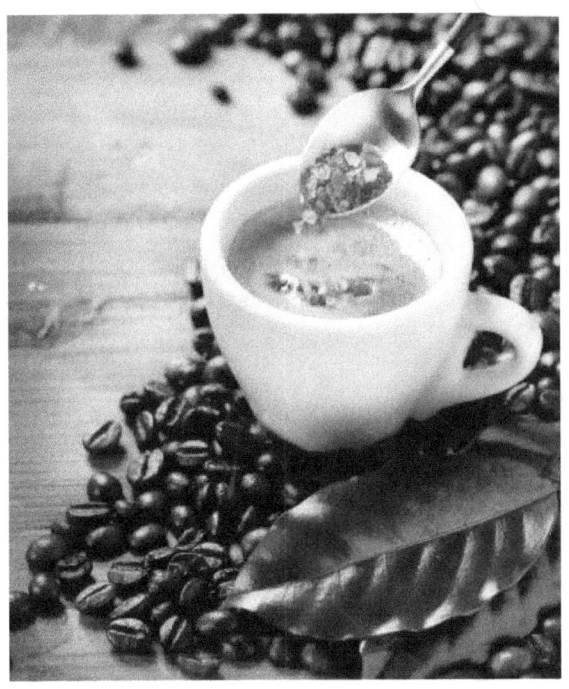

# Health Learning Series

### Dueep J. Singh

### Mendon Cottage Books

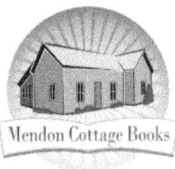

*JD-Biz Publishing*

**Disclaimer**

The information is this book is provided for informational purposes only. It is not intended to be used and medical advice or a substitute for proper medical treatment by a qualified health care provider. The information is believed to be accurate as presented based on research by the author.

The contents have not been evaluated by the U.S. Food and Drug Administration or any other Government or Health Organization and the contents in this book are not to be used to treat cure or prevent disease.

The author or publisher is not responsible for the use or safety of any diet, procedure or treatment mentioned in this book. The author or publisher is not responsible for errors or omissions that may exist.

**Warning**

The Book is for informational purposes only and before taking on any diet, treatment or medical procedure, it is recommended to consult with your primary health care provider.

Our books are available at

1. Amazon.com
2. Barnes and Noble
3. Itunes
4. Kobo
5. Smashwords
6. Google Play Books

# Table of Contents

# Introduction

Once upon a time, thousands of years ago an Ethiopian shepherd possibly in the Kaffa region of the southwestern part of Africa found all his sheep dining of the succulent fruit off a bush. The only problem with that was that the moment they had eaten those berries, they started to grow more frisky.

So he decided to experiment a little. There was this old ewe, almost on her last legs. So he fed her some of those brown berries, and then spend the whole day, trying to capture her.

He sat down on a rock and began to think. If this is the effect that these beans had on an old ewe, could it have a similar rejuvenating effect upon his own father? So he collected some of the berries, and asked his woman to brew them in water. This brew was then given to his old ailing father. And then the whole village spent the whole day trying to capture the father, who was under the influence of a caffeine high.

Naturally, the father came down with a bump after the high was over and was sick for the next week. However, the Ethiopians found that this berry been drunk in moderate quantities was enough to rejuvenate them and give them a kick. And so kafe from the Kaffa region or the beans of Coffea arabica, which was first indigenous but then was slowly and steadily spread all over the world became one of the most popular brews drunk by mankind after water and tea.

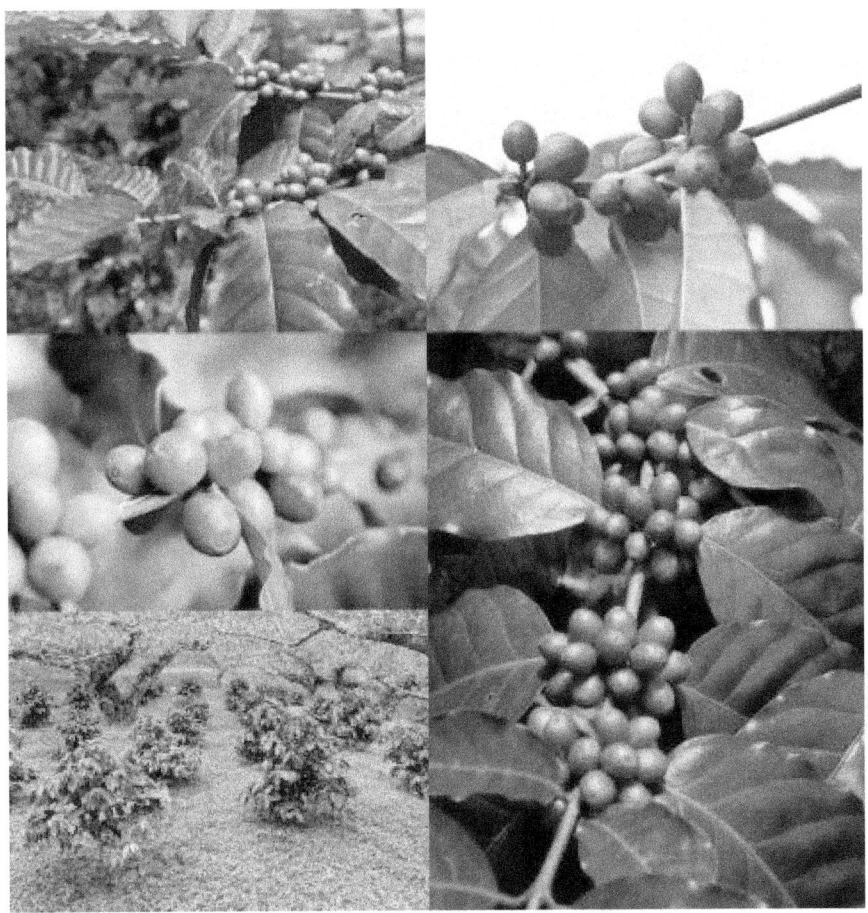

Use of coffee was introduced in the Mediterranean countries by the Arabs who spread this brew, in every country with which Arab traders were trading. In 575 A D, Coffee seeds were used in Yemen as recent acts, omissions show. The first record of Arabic work in which coffee was recorded was in 1454.

The use of coffee in Western Europe began around 1615, along with tea which arrived there around 1600 and cacao in 1525. So the cups of Java that you drink for breakfast or just for a stimulant are made up of about 60 species of the genus Coffea. Apart from Coffea arabica there are a number of African varieties grown for making coffee, but they are native and indigenous and grown in only a limited space and to a much smaller extent.

Out of these, C. liberica and C.canephora, which is also known as the robusta species is grown in all those areas where the original coffee Arabica cannot be grown easily. There was once a time when East Africa flourished with coffee plantations. These plantations always were made at high elevations, so that the flavor would be enhanced.

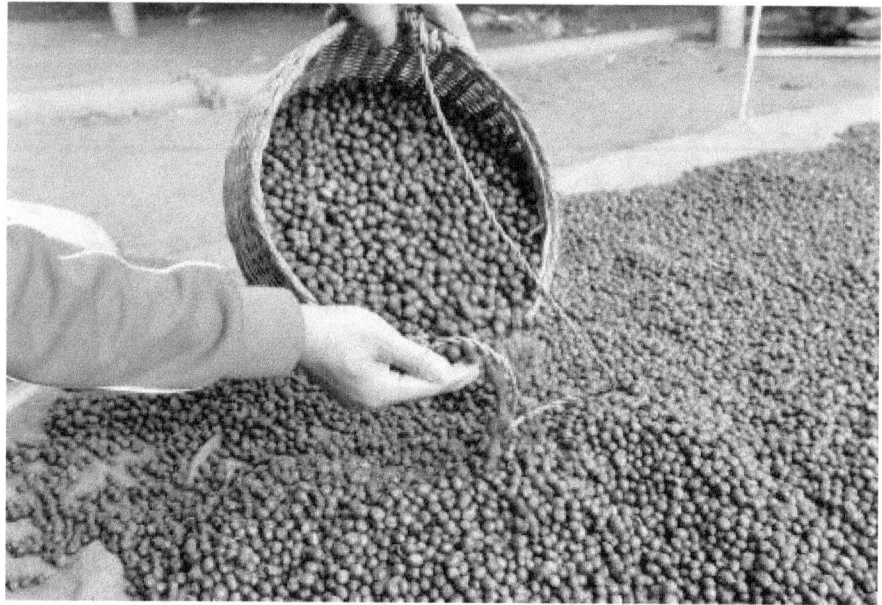

There is a wild species, which is known as C stenophylla. The fruit of this plant is normally collected from the wild plants and it is not cultivated.

The Gardenia belongs to the same family as coffee. So the flowers of the coffee plant are equally beautiful.

The top suppliers of coffee in the world is Brazil and Columbia. Coffee is also grown in other South American countries, as well as Central America, West Indies, East Africa and the Dutch East Indies.

In East Africa as well as in India, you can find clone varieties of coffee known as Kent and Jackson.

# Planting Coffee Trees

The shrubs of coffee can vary greatly in ultimate size, and you can also find little coffee trees about 14 feet tall to 30 feet. The coffee tree is going to have a strong dominant stem with horizontal, primary lateral branches in pairs opposite each other. These are now going to branch out to give paired secondary laterals. The secondary branches are going to form tertiary laterals which are going to be in one plane and at a right angle. The weight of the fruit and the leaves are going to cause these branches to droop.

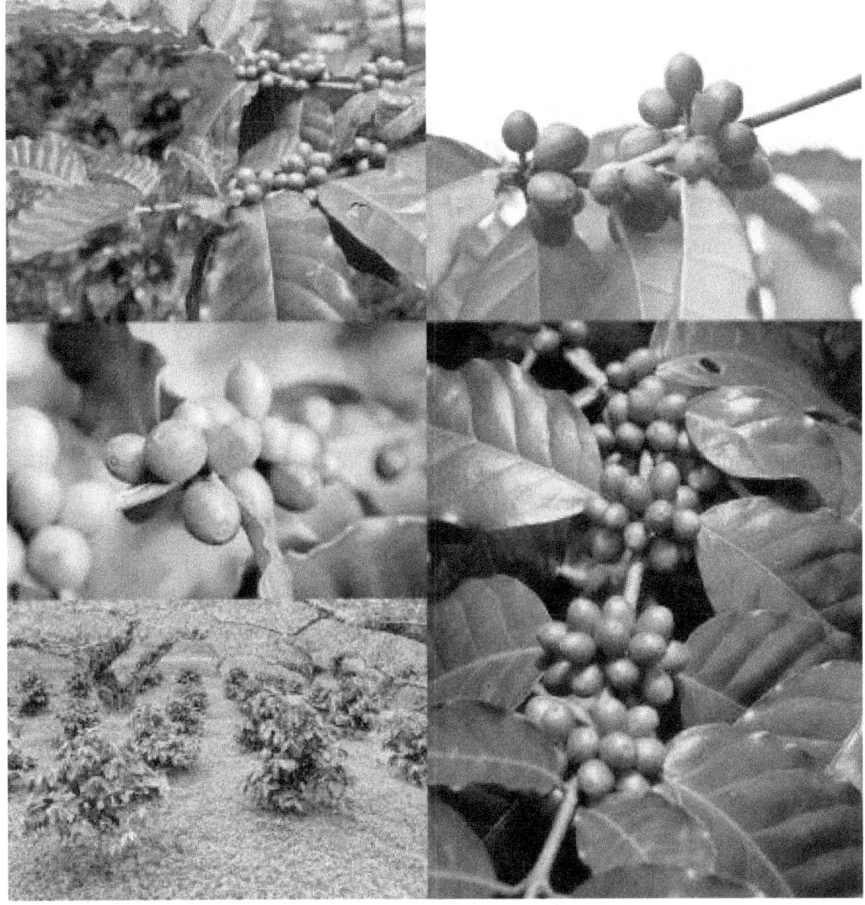

Although the tree is small, its early growth is rapid and it begins to fruit young, maybe bearing a considerable crop at four years and in full bearing

---

at six – seven years from the seed. In well fertilized and aerated soil, it may have many roots more than 4 feet deep.

Such rapid development of a tree that never becomes large, suggests a short-lived tree like that of the peach. However, coffee trees have been reported to live as long as 200 years, if insects or diseases and unfavorable environmental conditions do not shorten their lifetimes, and if the crops are not too heavy.

However, one coffee planting is going to be unprofitable after 20 – 40 crops.

The time of flowering in a coffee plant is going to depend on the climate if there is a rather long dry spell and the irrigation is not regular. Nearly all the flowers are going to open about a month after the rains have begun. These flowers are beautiful heavy and white blossoms, but their blossoming is going to be straggling.

However, if the moisture supply is good throughout the year, and there is time period of temperature too low for proper growth, the flowering as well as the maturing of the plant may be at a regular time periods throughout the whole year.

If there are several rather short periods of water stress during the year, relatively light flowering may follow each dry period. In Puerto Rico from flowering tends to be from February to June. Each flower is going to have a Corolla with five lobes curled in such a manner that the clumps of white flowers at each dark waxy green leaf in the pairs along the horizontal branches are strikingly beautiful.

# Fruit

The fruit is set thickly from the flowers that the pair of the leaves on the literal branches. The shoot of course is elongated beyond the flower clusters, while the fruit is growing. Flower buds on the New wood are not initiated until after the fruit is harvested if your coffee crop is heavy.

Not all of the flowers are going to set fruit. Records in Puerto Rico show that 26% of the flowers grew fruit, especially in West Indian seedling clones and varieties. Columnaris is a variety which gives you 16% of yield. The greater crops of this particular variety is because of a larger number of flowers on a tree.

The mature fruit can be almost disc shaped or slightly oblong about a half inch thick in diameter and somewhat more than a half inch long, red to nearly black. The time from blossom to a ripe fruit is about 6 to 7 months from the trees grown in Puerto Rico and just this little bit less for Blue Mountain Trees, especially if you are looking for February blossom, rather than the blossoms opening later, when the weather turns hotter.

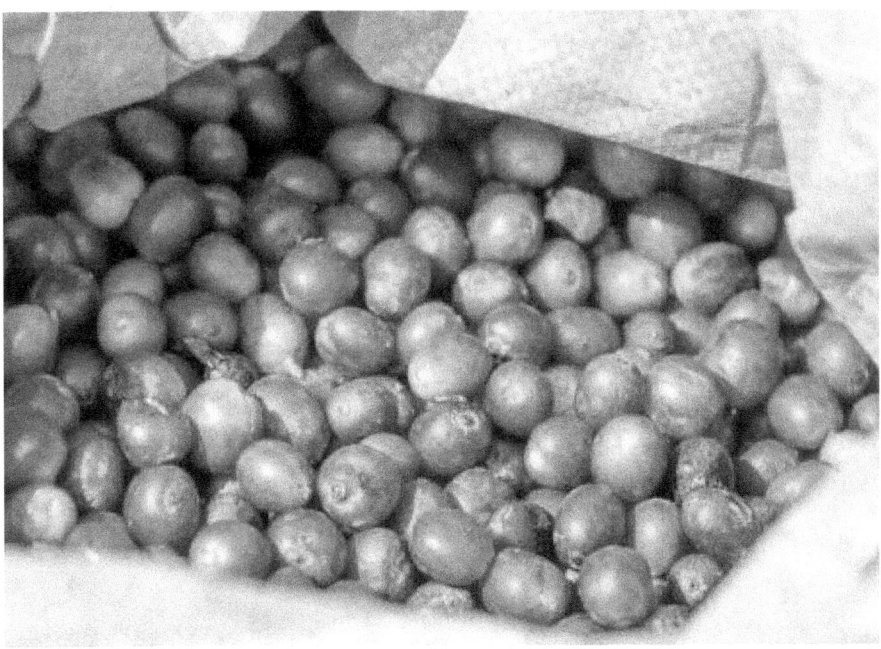

Fruits before the extraction of the seeds are usually called cherries. The yield of freshly harvested fruits are going to be called cherry yield.

This coffee fruit is sometimes called a drupe and sometimes called the coffee berry. It is going to differ in morphology from other groups like peach or cherry in having 2 seeds, each enclosed by a separate parchment and a hard endocarp.

The part of the fruit that is used is the seed. It has under the parchment a perisperm known as the Silver skin. This is formed from the tissue of the outer integument.

Apart from this the seed also has an endosperm which is much the largest part of the seed and probably contributes most to the cup of coffee. The embryo is going to have two small cotyledons.

The weight of the seed – coffee Bean – after the removal of the parchment and dried to the market requirement is going to be 13 – 17% of the weight of the whole fruit when it was harvested.

That is because the weight of the parchment – endocarp – is about 1/3 – 1/5 the weight of the dried bean.

This extra material was discarded until it was found that it was very rich in nitrogen, phosphorus and potassium. That is why it was returned back to the soil. It is also excellent in making vinegar because it is rich in carbohydrates. This experimentation started in Puerto Rico, but it did not extend to other places where coffee beans were grown regularly and in large quantities.

The yield of a dried bean per acre is going to be quite variable. That is because this is going to depend on the fruitfulness of the seedling, the variation in the soil and the climate and the coffee variety being grown.

Yield of different coffee plants have varied anywhere between 1200 pounds per acre per year – 542 pounds in other places. In Hawaii, especially the Kona area, the average yield per acre per year was 250 pounds!

That is why researchers on coffee yields believe that there is a tendency for yield in one year to be correlated with the amount of shoot growth made in the preceding year, because the fruit is borne on these particular shoots.

Unless the climate is one in which a prolonged dry period are some other influences cause very heavy blossoming in a short period, there will be green fruit of different ages on the trees at harvesting time. Only the seeds of the fruit ripened on the tree to a dark red cherry can be processed to good flavored beans.

Pickers are expected to select only such fruit and not to damage the green fruit.

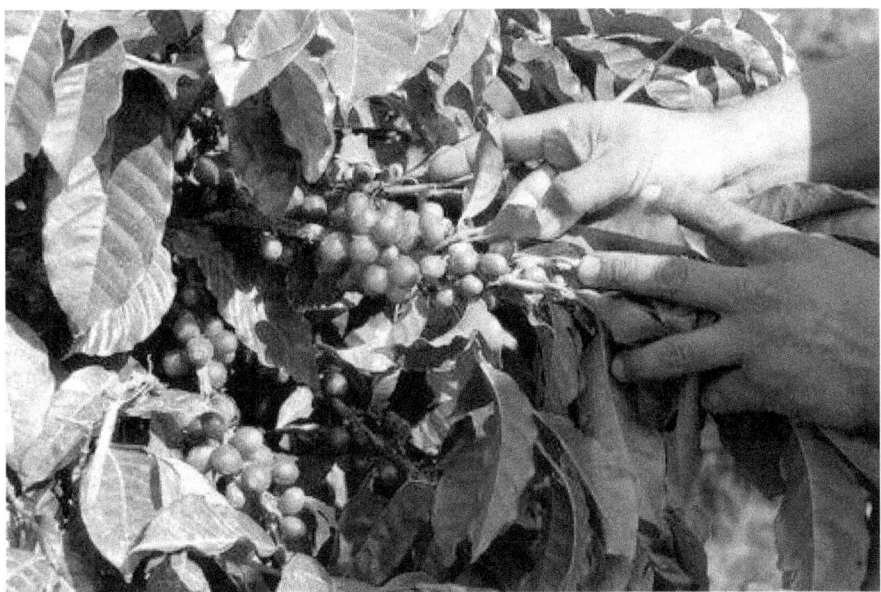

# Separation of the Exocarp and Misocarp

There are two general methods of separating the exocarp and the sticky misocarp from the beans. These are the dry and the wet methods.

By the dry method, the fruit is going to be spread about 3 inches deep on a drying pavement where it is going to be turned frequently. It is going to be gathered in heaps before night and protected from possible rain. After the seeds are nearly dry enough, they are piled in a heap and covered so that the final degree of dryness is uniform among all the seeds. These precautions, including the avoidance of exposure to rain is going to keep the green color in the coffee Bean.

The dried fruits may be stored several weeks to several months or you can hull them immediately.

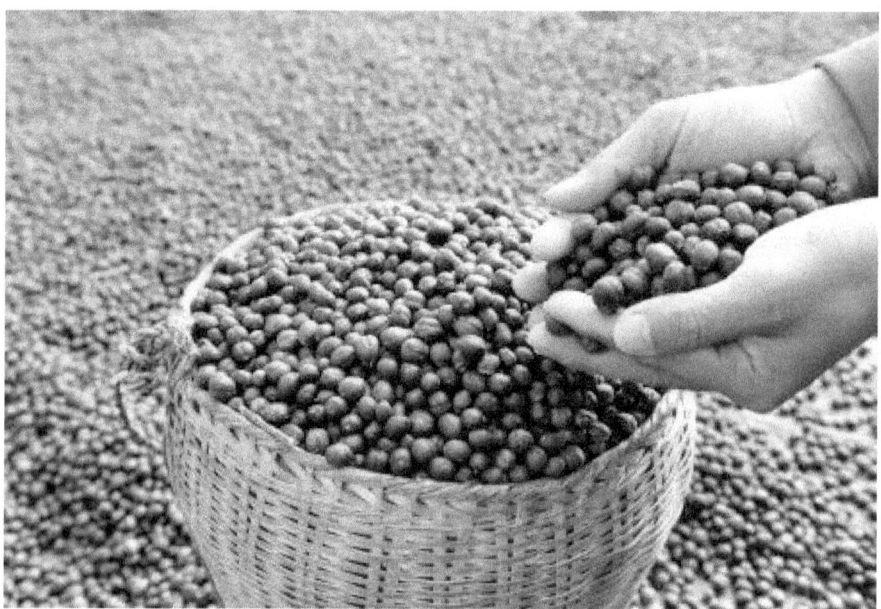

# Hulling

Hulling is the removal of exocarp, mesocarp and endocarp with a pestle and mortar. This has been done traditionally in this manner for thousands of years, but nowadays, hulling machines are used extensively, especially on coffee plantations.

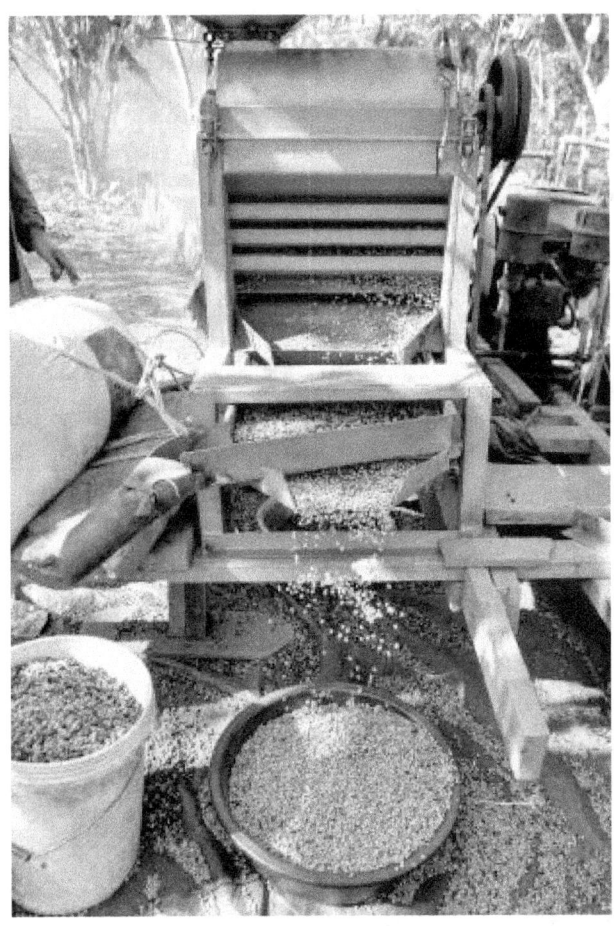

Use of the dry method for Arabica coffee is satisfactory, only in a region where humidity of the air, and the rainfall during the harvesting is too low for much development of dry rot and molds.

In such a climate, the coffee, cleaned by the dry method is going to be of good quality and on a par with the coffee dried by the wet method. Artificial dryers are now being tried out in many places all over the world, for more complete control over drying processes.

The mesocarp, also known as the flesh of the seed is less succulent and it does not get much injured by humidity during the drying process.

By the wet method, the cherries are going to be held for a night in water to soften the skin. They can also be floated directly into hoppers of pulping machines. This is going to remove the exocarp and as much of the mesocarp as possible.

The seeds are then run into tanks of water and left until the fermentation process makes the sticky fleshy material more easily removable. This change seems to be due largely to an enzyme in the fruit. However, bacteria and yeasts are also capable of hastening the fermentation process.

The action of the bacteria is going to hasten the action by increasing the acidity of the material to a reaction more favorable for the activity of the enzyme. But this supposedly worked process, aided by the bacteria may cause too much of acidity in the beans. This is known as foxiness!

Fermentation process for 16 – 48 hours is adequate, especially if the temperature is low.

In Central American countries, peptic enzymes were added to the liquid to reduce this, to anywhere between 4 to 6 hours. In Kenya, no concentration of the enzyme reduced this to 12 hours. However, that lowered the quality of the coffee. Quick method experiments were done because they would reduce the loss of weight by fermentation in the coffee bean. However, if you are willing to compromise up the quality of the coffee as an end product, you may try out these quick fermentation methods.

After fermentation, the coffee is washed with adequate stirring to remove the loosened fleshy material and dried for a number of days spread on the pavement or you can dry it for a considerably shorter time in the special dryer.

It is then run through appealing machine to remove the parchment. It can now be run at once or later through a machine to remove the silvery skin and polish the beans. These are now graded for size so that the length of the roasting can be accurately adjusted for best quality.

Coffee processed by the wet method is going to have better flavor and is thus more expensive.

# Flavor of the Coffee

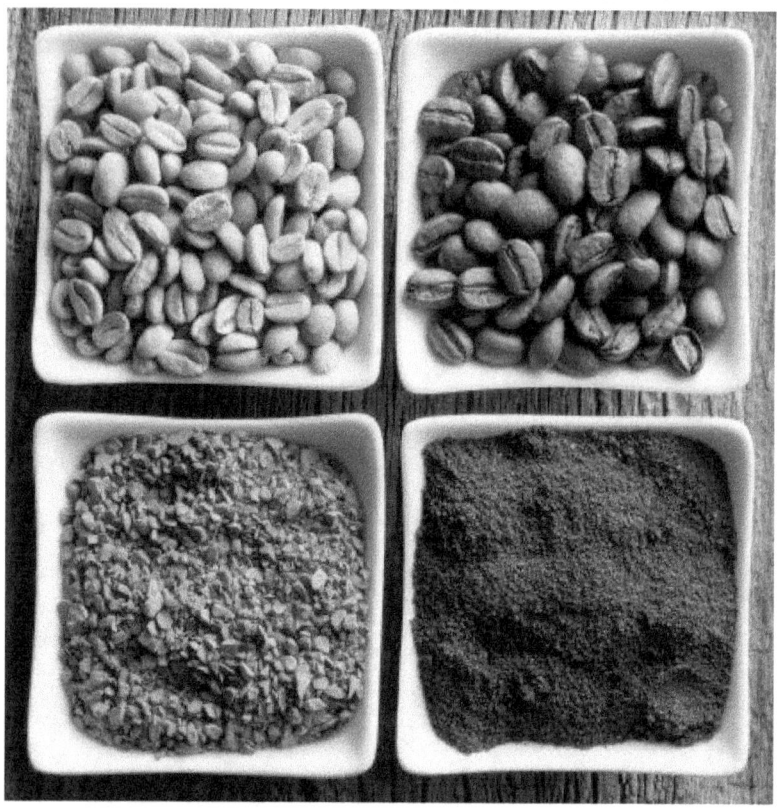

**Green coffee, ground coffee, roasted coffee and instant coffee**

The flavor of the coffee is of course going to be influenced greatly by the method of making it. Boiling, for example, is going to bring on a bitter flavor. A grind finer than that normally used is going to make a better drink.

I do not drink tea or coffee. But when I used to stay with my friends in South India, I was woken up every morning with the delicious aroma of freshly ground coffee beans, which had been roasted fresh. It is a tradition in many parts of India that the new bride is requested to make two things when she enters the in-laws house for the first time. The first is a sweet dish – rice pudding – and the second one is coffee, especially in South India.

If she makes coffee perfectly, it is considered that her mother taught her all the domestic sciences well! Ground coffee, which is packed in vacuum cans are going to lose flavor faster. The lower the vacuum at which is packed is going to slow down the loss of flavor. So a vacuum of about 29 inches is good for packing coffee. But in many parts of the East, vacuum packed coffee is considered to be anathema. Also in South America. Fresh coffee beans which you need to roast and grind by yourself and bring down fresh is the best way to start the day for millions all over the world.

Coffee Arabica is going to have a much better flavor than any other robusta forms. And a better drink is going to be made from this coffee grown at higher elevations than at lower elevations.

Coffees are blended to suit the varied tastes of the American market. All of them are not exactly from the high or low elevations, but they are mixed to make a blend.

Coffee grown at the elevations above 5000 – 6000 feet, may be too acid for the best flavor, if used alone, but they are excellent for blending. Other influences determining the taste and flavor of the coffee is going to be the health of the tree and the care taken in processing, which is going to affect the ultimate flavor.

The blend and each constituent of the resulting brew is normally tested by professionals, trained and selected to detect undesirable odors and flavors in their cup of Java .

The stimulant in coffee is caffeine, but other substances are also going to give the flavors which determine the price in discriminating markets. Knowledge of these substances are really not known yet, but we know that there is a N – methyl betaine part of nicotinic acid, which is known as trigonalline. The pleasant bitter flavor that you taste, as a pleasant sensation to the lips, the moment you drink your cup of coffee is known as acid.

The difference in degree of this acidic sensation given can hardly be due to different in hydrogen ion concentration in the solution. That is because all the coffees – the poorest and the best – fall between the pH range of 4.9 – 5.3.

# Growing Coffea Arabica

Arabica coffee is normally grown at 3500 – 6500 feet elevation, or a little higher. This is known in the coffee trade as mild coffee from which you can get a better drink when compared to the coffee of the same variety grown at a lower elevation.

Coffee, which is grown at a lower elevation is known as harsh coffee. Robusta species and Liberica are also going to give you better yield and flavor when they are grown at higher elevation, but not so good that you can put them in a class with Arabica coffee.

The beneficial effect on quality may be due to a lower temperature at a higher elevation as seen in the Kona region in Hawaii.

## Temperature –

The leaves of Arabica trees seem to be a little more resistant to frost than those of other tropical plants like bananas. However, the tree has less ability than some others to produce new shoots after a frost, which has killed all the leaves and has damaged the wood.

Such a tree is going to be tolerant of cool summers and less tolerant of very high summer temperatures than many other tropical species like banana, papaya, and cacao. And less resistant to frost and too high summer temperatures when compared to tea plants.

## Shade –

Much of the coffee grown in the world is grown in the shade of larger trees of other species. In some situations, the shade may cause some improvement in the flavor of drink that is made from coffee seeds.

Excellent coffee can be grown without shade at higher elevations. However, in areas where the temperature is quite high, the sky is not hazy or foggy, and the sunlight is intense, coffee trees thrive best in partial shades. This is what is being done in Brazil , Kona and East Africa, when the best results are without shade, but the soil is well covered with a mulch.

The blue Mountains yield in East Africa is reported not to fruit as well, and then stared as some other coffee farms grown there. Photosynthesis and the growth of the coffee trees have been found a little more rapid under full sunlight. The growth of coffee trees have been found a little more rapid under partial shade than in full sunlight. This is possibly in part because of the stomata closing earlier in the day in full sunlight.

The leaves in dense shade however, such as those in the center of dense trees are much slower in photosynthesis, than leaves in sunlight. In Puerto Rico, yield, and the growth of the trees are increase significantly by artificial shade that reduce the light on the coffee trees to about half of full sunlight.

The best trees that provide the right amount of shade for growing coffee plants are tall trees like Cassie, Inga, Erythrina and Albizzia.

These are tree species which supply their own nitrogen. Any tree which is going to root deeper than a coffee tree and obtain much of their water below the root level of the coffee tree is going to be an excellent shade tree.

If you plant a species that is best when the soil is deep enough for this is going to weaken the coffee trees in soil so shallow that all the roots are going to compete with the coffee roots.

Sometimes in regions where the water supply is not enough for both shade trees and coffee, dense row of tall trees on the windward side of a considerable block is going to lift the dry wind and improve the health of the coffee trees without competition with many of them for water.

## Water –

As is logical, any water deficit that reduces the growth of the tree in one year is going reduce the crop in the succeeding year.

## Soil

If the rainfall is adequate and frequent the coffee tree is going to be tolerant of shallow and somewhat impervious soils in deep salt, however the roots of the young trees are going to penetrate to a greater depth rapidly.

If the trees must survive for rather longer periods without rainfall such a large root system in deep soil needs to be essential for good growth and production.

Coffee trees seem to find a soil reaction between pH 7 more favorable but they – compared to tea trees who prefer acid soils – find a little bit of lime added to the soil, if the pH value is around 4.7 pH to be more beneficial.

Too much of lime added to the soil is going to cause chlorosis in the plant.

## Soil erosion

Being grown at a high elevation, often on rather steep slopes and where the rainfall is apt to be heavy plantations that reduce coffee of the best quality are often subject to serious losses by soil erosion. In some parts of the world, some land has been planted that apparently could not be protected by any treatment that the crops could ever pay for. That was because the blocks of several terraces could go out at any time. However the roots of the coffee trees and the shade trees help to hold the soil together and leaving low growing needs between the trees can help prevent soil erosion.

In Kenya, coffee plantations have mulches of elephant grass or other materials, such as maize, or sorghum stalks applied just before the time of the long rains, so that there is minimal soil erosion and consequently the yield of the coffee improves a lot.

Mulches can be used in building terraces where the slopes are not steep at planting silt basins may be dug into each space between plants along the row. The soil has to be thrown along the middle below the rows. Mulch material can be piled on this and the soil that washes into the silt basins can then be thrown on to the mulch after the rains. Eventually rather good terraces can be formed in this way, providing the tree rows follow the contours well or fairly well.

If you are growing coffee in steeper land with complicated slope, the contours for the rows should be run by professional surveyors. The decision concerning the wisdom of planting in such a location should thus be based in part of that professional advice who has been studying soil erosion problems in such a situation carefully and for a long time.

If the rains are not too heavy, mulches are going to reduce erosion by keeping the soil surface highly permeable to water so that more of the rainfall enters the soil instead of running off the surface. Even the falling leaves and the pruning from coffee trees and leaves from the shade trees are going to help in this.

If the rainfall is in a number of light showers and the total required is barely adequate, this increased permeability of the soil surface is going to add considerably to the water supply for the trees by causing penetration instead of a runoff.

In East Africa, this increased penetration of water caused by a mulch applied before the beginning of an inadequate rainy season benefited the coffee trees more than the reduced evaporation from the soil surface caused by a mulch applied at the ending of a rainy season.

Trampling of the soil at harvesting fruit and caring for the trees tends to reduce its surface permeability, unless a mulch, or a low growth of plants protects the surface.

Remember that cultivation of any type is going to compact the soil, but it is also going to increase the coffee yield during the first few years at least, if the rainfall is inadequate to supply water for both weeds and the coffee trees.

In many parts of Kenya, where the annual rainfall varies from anywhere between 25 – 54 inches, 30-year-old coffee trees had their yield reduced to 39% by the free growth of weeds and 27% by weeds kept low by slashing. The plots which did not have any weeds at all gave the most yield.

# Necessary Nutrients for Coffee Growth

By preventing soil and sheet erosion, the mulch which holds the part of the soil that is apt to be the richest in highly available nutrients, especially nitrogen and of course mulch disintegration is going to supply all the nutrients required by the plant any nutrient deficiency can be reduced by regular applications of nitrogen and motivation as well as phosphorus. In the Kona region of Hawaii, coffee trees are not going to yield well unless you apply potassium to them.

A nitrogen deficiency is going to be seen by a yellowing of leaves somewhat like that in lime induced chlorosis. Apply lots of nitrogen and this yellowing is going to go away. Milder symptoms of nitrogen deficiency, such as reduced growth and light/pale color of the foliage may show in a growth flush made during the rainy season owing to the leaching out of the nitrate nitrogen from the soil.

So if you are a serious coffee grower, how are you going to determine the fertilizing needs of your trees, taking into view, different seedling trees and different mountain soils? For this you need to get a leaf analysis done by a professional. For example, one such study showed that as much as seven plots of 20 trees each received one particular treatment. They were then compared with as many trees without the treatment in order to be reasonably certain that an apparent increase in yield of 20% was actually due to the treatment and not due to the accidental superiority of the trees or the soil of the treated plots.

Deficiencies of manganese, zinc, and even boron are considered to be serious among coffee growers in many parts of Central America. Spraying equipment is quite hard to haul over these uneven areas so a soil application has to be done by hand.

# Enemies of Coffee

Apart from the birds and the other pests attacking the ripening coffee berries during harvest time, there are other enemies of. There are some leaf blights which are caused by fungus. Some diseases are caused by insects. In the 19th century, the Arabica coffee growth in Ceylon, Indonesia and Philippines was nearly wiped out due to one of these fungal diseases. That is why the Robusta species was introduced here.

An abundant nitrogen supply and vigorous growth is going to increase the resistance of the plants. You can spray the plants with copper compounds to control any sort of fungal infection.

Many areas where coffee is grown as a powerful economic crop, there are plenty of researchers who know all about the diseases and the insects of local importance, which may harm your yield. Close planting and uneven mountain land often makes getting through with proper and efficient control equipment very difficult and also very expensive. Some places have been suffering from a chronic and serious root disease problem, and that means that the coffee growers have to do a continuous replacement program periodically or continuously, depending on the virulence of the disease.

# Growing of Coffee Trees

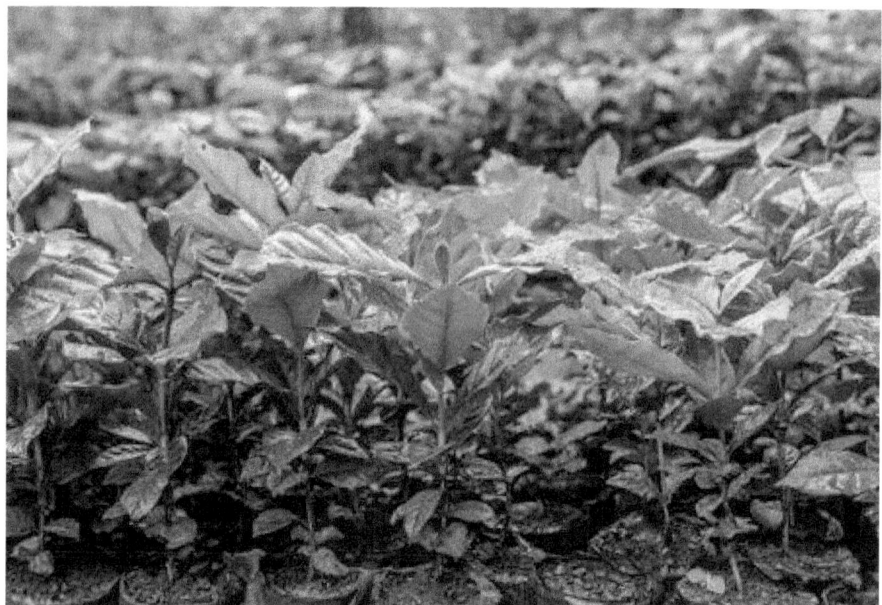

The normal way to grow coffee trees is done by vegetative propagation in the form of leafy cuttings. **These cuttings have to be made of upright stem branches. They should never be from the spreading lateral branches.** Such lateral branch cuttings are going to root but they are going to produce only spreading branches along the ground.

If you want to produce leafy cuttings *only* from a tree, plant, the parent tree in a nursery row and train it to multiple stems. Plant these trees 5 feet apart.

When the plant is large enough – about 24 months old – you can now pegged down the stems to horizontal positions and cut off the laterals.

The new upright shoots are going to grow from just below where the laterals were attached. All of these can be taken for cuttings except three of them at good positions for new stems to supply future cuttings for you after they have been pegged down.

The cuttings are best taken when the wood has begun to show partial hardening at the base. The succulent apex has to be discarded to where 2 good leaves can be left attached.

In fact, single node cuttings with stem projection below the two leaf node far enough for planting have given extremely good results.

## Rooting –

Leaves on the part above the ground are highly important for good rooting and growth after rootings. In East Africa the best potting medium used was coarse sand mixed with twice the amount of peat moss. In other parts of the world coarse sand and coconut fiber in equal quantities give equally good results. However, in Puerto Rico, they just use coarse sand.

Direct sunlight should not reach the cuttings. Humidity must be maintained at nearly 90%. This means that you will need to put on a glass cover on the propagating frame to admit light, but which is going to impede the escape of moisture. Frequent light spraying of the cuttings or a continuous mist throughout the sunniest spot of the day also helps in better cutting growth.

This high humidity and the reduced light is necessary to prevent any sort of abscission of the leaves. A regular temperature of about 70° to 75°F is best for their growth.

Good drainage in the rooting medium also is very important. You will need to put in a thick layer of rocks graded from the largest at the bottom to the smallest just under the rooting medium and still small enough to hold this medium in place.

Coffee cuttings are sensitive plants! Even such a minor detail as wrapping shoots taken in the field with a wet cloth to avoid the smallest amount of wilting in taking them to the propagating frames or making a fresh basal cut at planting seems to have a significant influence on the percentage to root.

This rooting process is rather slow, beginning at 2 ½ months to three months after setting. 75% may be rooted in four – six months. A few may still yet be alive and beginning to root after two years if they are left there that long!

The base of a cutting may show a ring of callus around it in five or six weeks after the cutting is set.

After the cuttings have been potted into a rich compost they are returned for three – four weeks to the humid frames. They are then held for two or three months in the shade without humidity control to harden before being planted in the nursery row, under some shade.

However, nowadays, many of the coffee trees that are planted are seedlings. This ceiling selection is done to maintain or improve the performance of the seedling form grown in that particular area. The seeds are selected from superior trees and groups of seedlings from each such tree are isolated so that the pollination is done from within the group.

Seedlings from these are fairly uniform in showing the merits of their parent trees.

Coffee seeds are durable and they can be kept in a cool place in sand for several months. The pulp is removed from them, but the parchment – endocarp – is left on. Seeds are usually planted in nursery beds under the shade, about 3 inches apart in a row and about a half inch deep, where they germinate in 6 to 7 weeks if the soil is kept moist.

When the seeds are about 8 inches tall, they are set about 12 inches apart in new nursery rows from which they are taken to the orchard after about 18 months or so. Sometimes the seeds may be planted further apart, and the seedlings taken to the orchard from the first nursery bed.

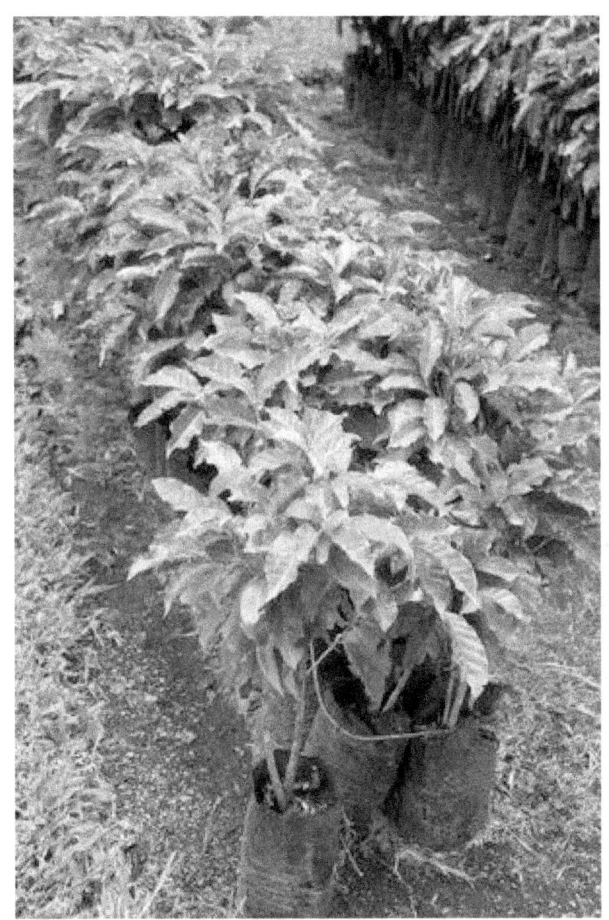

# Planting

In Guatemala, interest is being shown in Hedgerow planting. That means the steep slopes are going to be covered with single row hedges about 10 feet apart on control terraces with the trees 3 feet apart in the hedges.

On gentler slopes a hedge can be composed of two or three rows with the hedges farther apart. Little pruning may be done and when the trees begin to decline in the yield new hedges are planted in the wide strips between the old hedges.

In traditional practices trees were set 9 feet apart each way in contours if the land was really rather deep and broad holes were made, sometimes as much as 24 in.$^2$ and 18 – 24 inches deep. These were dug some weeks before the planting time. They were then allowed to weather. After that they were filled a little more than levels fall with topsoil mixed with rotting organic manure.

A new hole of convenient size was then made in this area where the tree was planted.

In some plantations in Brazil, good seed beds are prepared in these holes and 15 – 20 seeds are planted in each of them. These young seedlings that grow are then thinned out, 4 – 6 seeds at each tree position. Such groups are now going to be treated as single trees.

If the nursery soil has enough of clay to hold a ball of soil and earth around the roots, the trees may withstand transplanting a little better if they are dug up in this way. However, in humid weather, coffee trees can withstand bare root transplanting quite well.

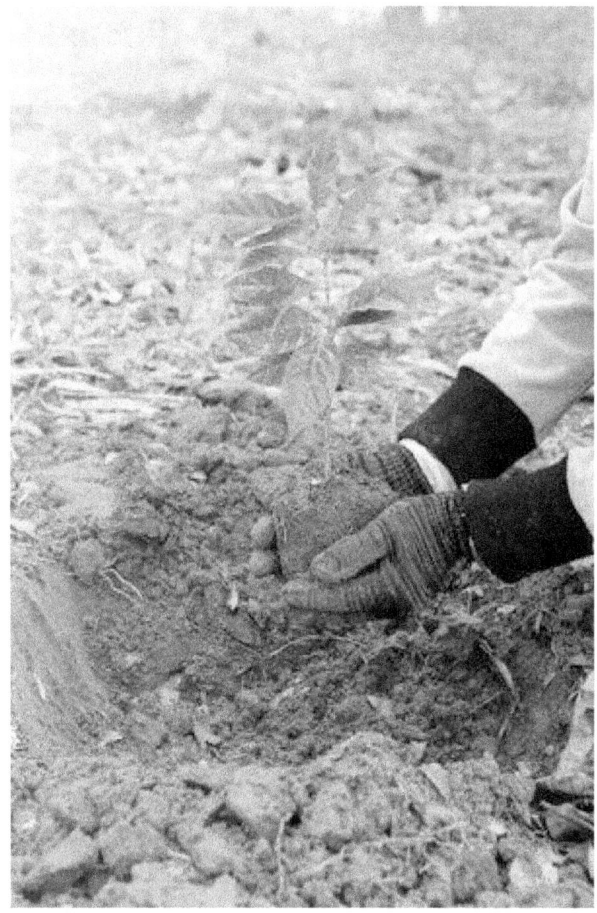

In areas where the weather may be unfavorable at any planting time, the young trees are grown in containers made of material that does not have to be removed for planting, but is going to disintegrate in the soil.

## Harvesting

Coffee pickers normally use one hand to hold the branches down – those within reach, – before picking off the fruit. In some places a picker may use a hook with a length of cord attached so that the branch is pulled downwards slowly by the hook and then attached at a convenient place. This is now held down by the cord wrapped around his foot, so that he can use both hands for picking.

# Making Coffee – one  Traditional Way

Believe it or not, quarrels about how to make coffee, the best way have been hotter than political dissertations and discussions or support for football and soccer teams.

The coffee, which I woke up to, when I was staying with my South Indian friends, is commonly known as filter Kapi. It is made out of roasted beans. And this is the way you make it. The beans which are commonly used here are coffee Arabica. Along with that you need a coffee filter. This is going to create a really delicious brew to which sugar and hot milk is added.

This milky coffee is going to have 70% – 80% of coffee beans which have been roasted. To this one adds 20% – 30% of chicory.

This coffee is made by putting exactly the right amount of the ground coffee powder – filter coffee – following up with boiling hot water. This hot water is going to allow the rich coffee flavor to become a thick decoction of the proper consistency.

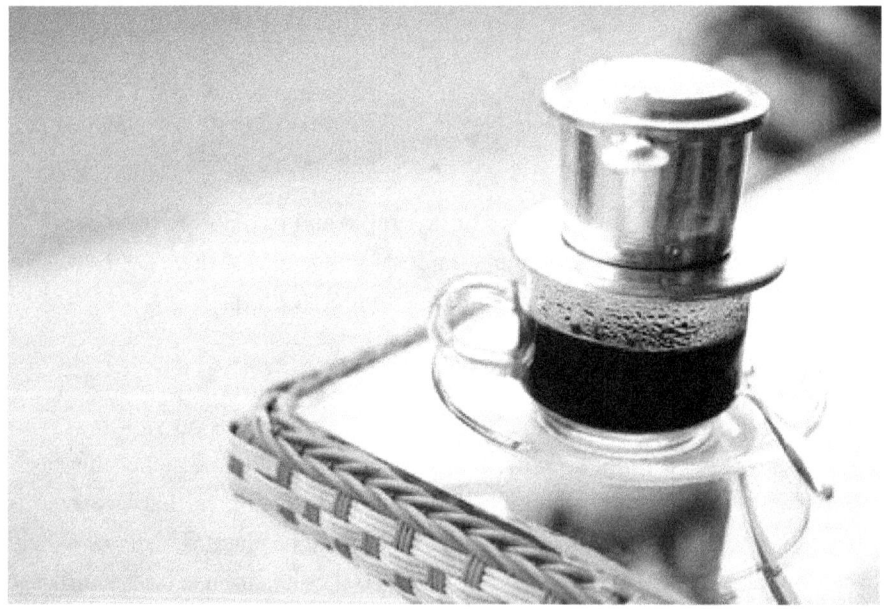

A typical coffee filter is going to be made up of three parts. The lowest chamber is where the coffee is collected after filtration, the topmost chamber is where the coffee powder, or the grounds are spooned and in which you poured the boiling water. There is also going to be a plunger which is going to be put in the uppermost portion, after the coffee, but before you pour in the water. All this is covered with a lid

The filter is perforated with two chambers – the upper and the lower. You put the coffee powder into the upper chamber. Cover this with the plunger. Now pour in the boiling water. Close the lid. This decoction is now going to drip into the lower portion. It may take anywhere between an hour or so, depending on the amount of water you put in. This is strong and thick. You can add more boiling water and go in for a second decoction which is going to be weaker.

Wait for an hour, you may say? That is not possible. I have to catch the 9 o'clock office goers rush. Well, you can set up this boiling water and coffee powder concoction in the coffee filter, just before you go to sleep. By the time you wake up you are going to have coffee ready at hand. Heat, add milk and sugar and drink. This decoction can be put in the fridge to be drunk throughout the day.

## Precautions

Do not heat this decoction, after you have added milk to the coffee. Remember to add this decoction to the heated sugar and milk, and not otherwise. This is going to tell you how much of decoction, you need so that you can get your cup of Java , well in time for the morning rush.

A decoction needs anywhere between three – four heaped tablespoons full of the coffee powder of your choice and boiling water.

Spoon the coffee powder into a dry and clean coffee filter. Do not tamp or pack it down, cover it with the plunger.

Pour the boiling water in until you fill up the upper chamber. Close this with the lid and leave the coffee to its own percolation.

For 1 cup of milky coffee, you need 2/3 cups of hot boiled milk and 3 tablespoons full of the first decoction. If you are using the second decoction which has been expressed, you will need about 1/3 cups of this liquid.

Sugar for tasting.

There is rather a bit of showmanship done in the making of this coffee, especially in South Indian restaurants. The coffee which is made from this process is known as Meter Coffee because the froth is obtained by pouring the coffee from a height of 1 m into a coffee tumbler which is placed in a utensil known as the dabara!

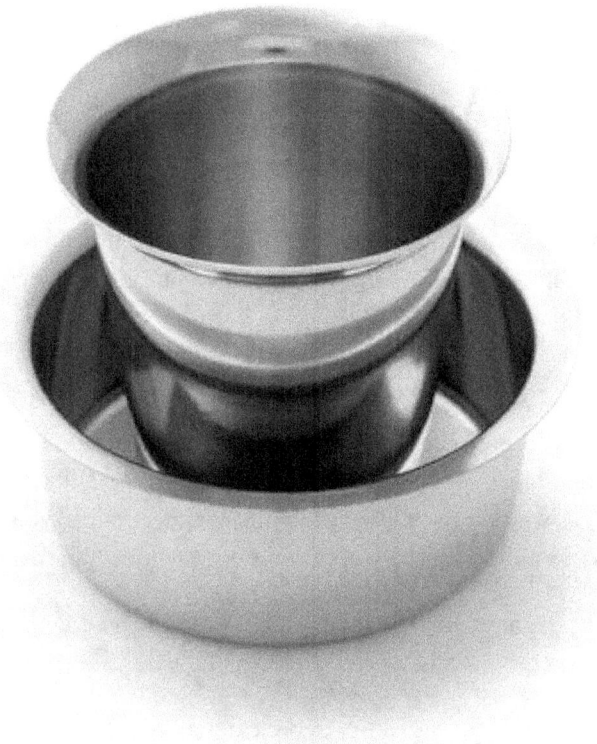

The milk is poured into a utensil, and then sugar and the decoction added to it. Then make it frothy by pouring it between two glasses, back and forth. Now one asks why the meter height is chosen for the pouring of this liquid, apart from it, making it frothy. The answer is very simple. The temperature is cooled down, so that you can sip it without burning your mouth.

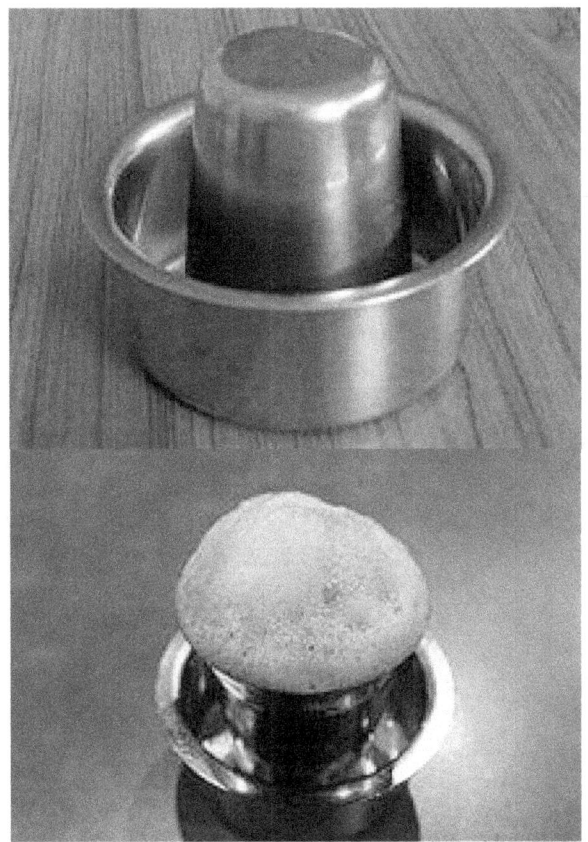

Image source : en.wikipedia.org Free Commons License

If you still find the coffee unbearably hot, your host or the restaurant or is going to pour it into the dabara. Contact with the metal is going to cool it down until the needed temperature is obtained. This coffee is also known as ½ kapi , which means two people can share it. One wants boiling hot coffee and the other gets cooled coffee. Elementary!

# Conclusion

This book gives you a deep insight into the life and times of coffee which is one stimulating drink without which many of us cannot do. That is not only because of its stimulating caffeine content, but also its addictive nature. So many of you are going to agree with that, if you have been reading this book while drinking your morning, afternoon or evening brew of coffee.

Doctors say that the use of stimulants like coffee, tea and cocoa are harmful to your health, and they are right because an excess of any item is going to be harmful to your health. So as long as you do not drink 20 cups of coffee[1] everyday, you will be all right! However, I would suggest not drinking too strong a brew, even if you **have** to gulp it down five times a day.

So enjoy your cup of java , Live Long and Prosper.

---

[1] Seen that in one of my more highly strung colleagues. She could not function without a couple of coffee and was soon prey to a myriad host of ailments like heart disease, ulcers, and other ailments. But then I think the ulcers were brought about by her worrywart nature because she would begin to start worrying about a project much before it came into reality or even took off, drinking coffee, all the while.

# Author Bio

**Dueep Jyot Singh** is a Management and IT Professional who managed to gather Postgraduate qualifications in Management and English and Degrees in Science, French and Education while pursuing different enjoyable career options like being an hospital administrator, IT,SEO and HRD Database Manager/ trainer, movie , radio and TV scriptwriter, theatre artiste and public speaker, lecturer in French, Marketing and Advertising, ex-Editor of Hearts On Fire (now known as Solstice) Books Missouri USA, advice columnist and cartoonist, publisher and Aviation School trainer, ex-moderator on Medico.in, banker, student councilor ,travelogue writer ... among other things!

One fine morning, she decided that she had enough of killing herself by Degrees and went back to her first love -- writing. It's more enjoyable! She already has 48 published academic and 14 fiction- in- different- genre books under her belt.

When she is not designing websites or making Graphic design illustrations for clients , she is browsing through old bookshops hunting for treasures, of which she has an enviable collection – including R.L. Stevenson, O.Henry, Dornford Yates, Maurice Walsh, De Maupassant, Victor Hugo, Sapper, C.N. Williamson, "Bartimeus" and the crown of her collection- Dickens "The Old Curiosity Shop," and so on... Just call her "Renaissance Woman" ) - collecting herbal remedies, acting like Universal Helping Hand/Agony Aunt, or escaping to her dear mountains for a bit of exploring, collecting herbs and plants and trekking.

Check out some of the other JD-Biz Publishing books

Gardening Series on Amazon

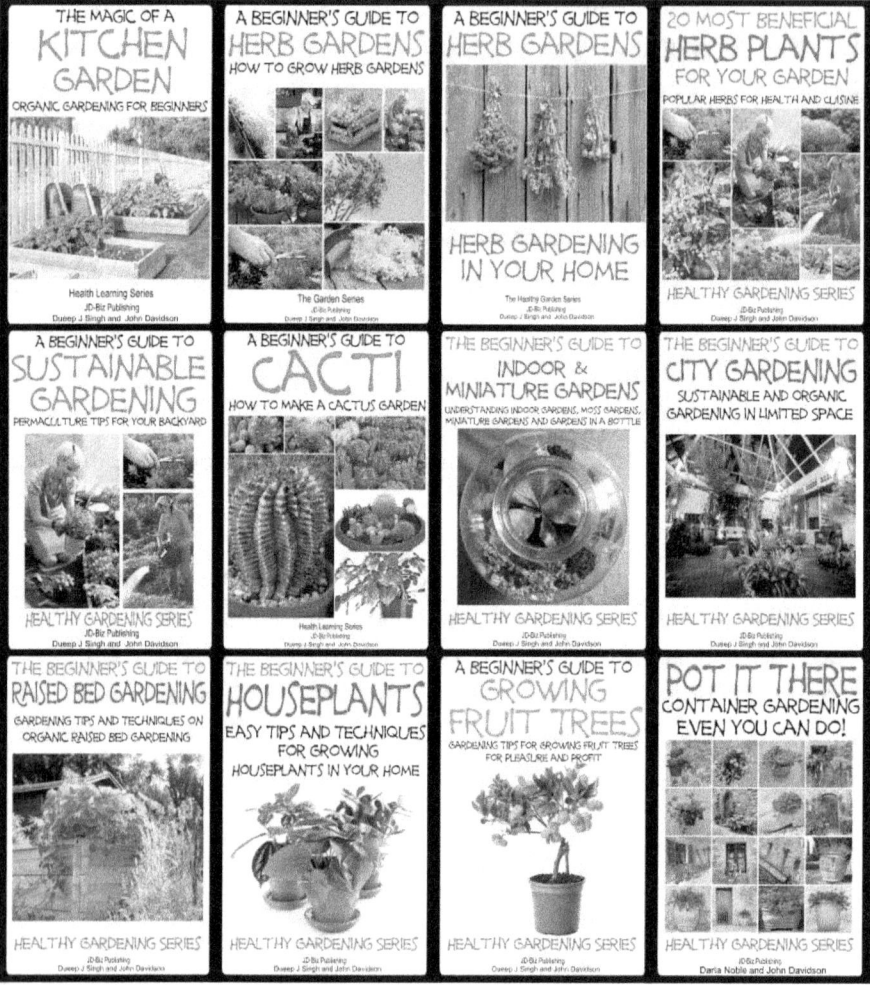

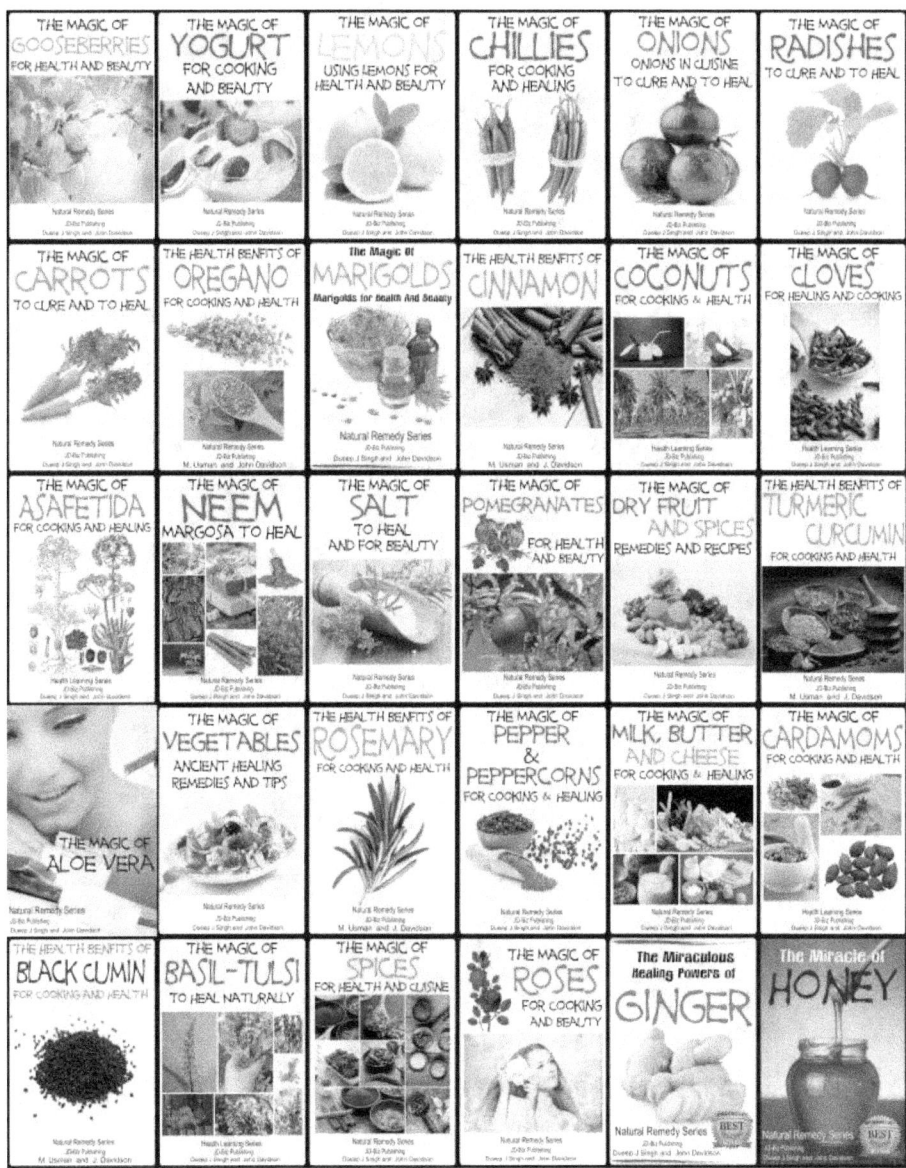

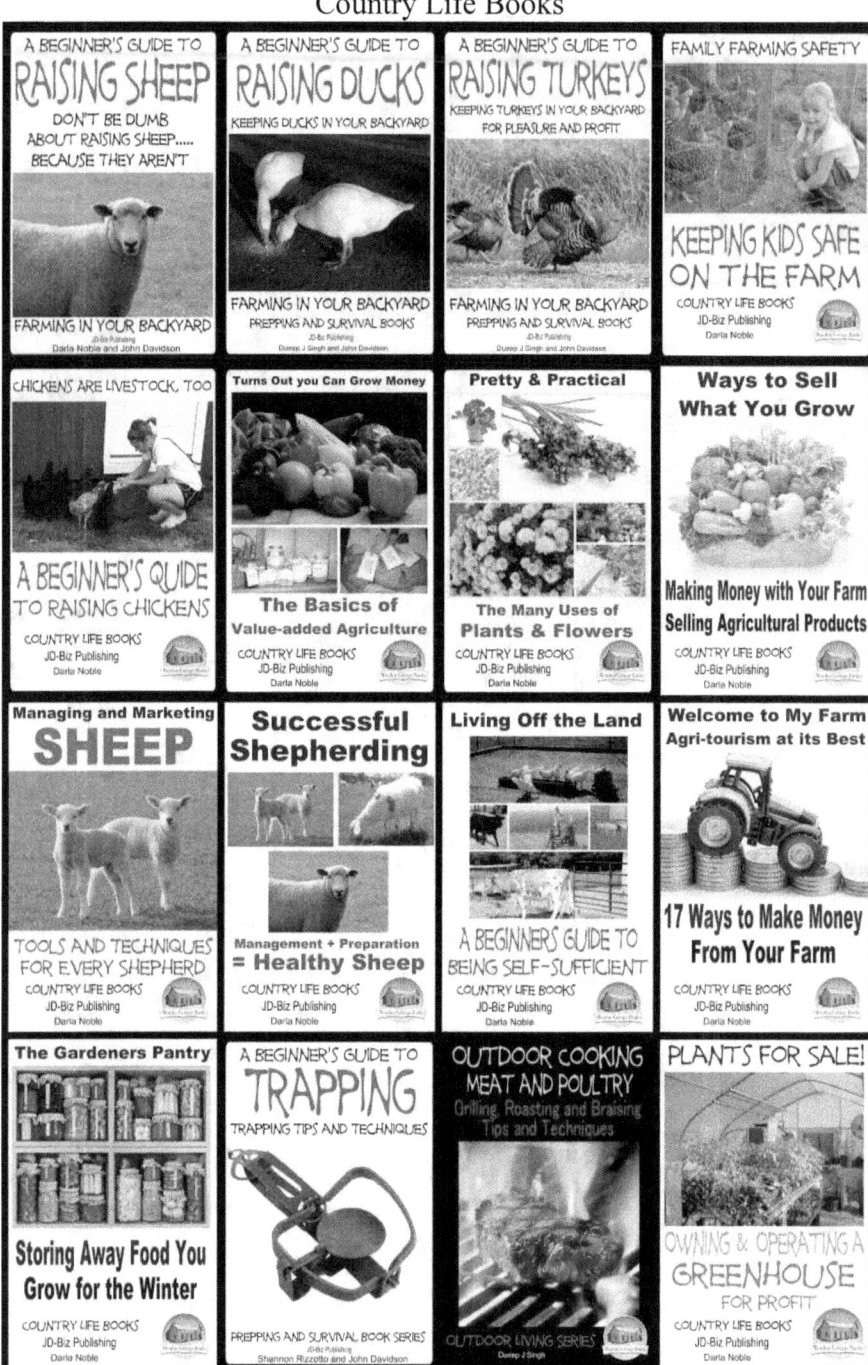

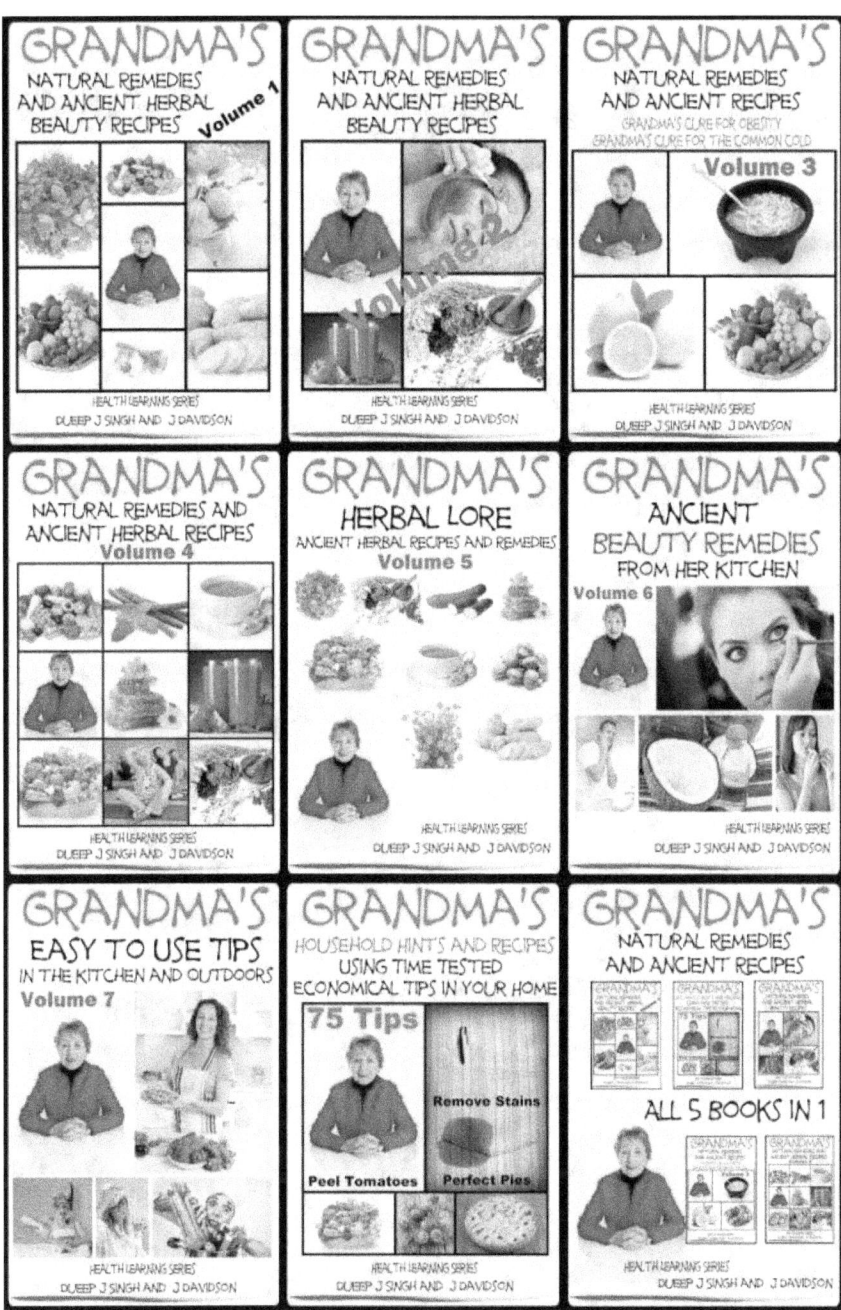

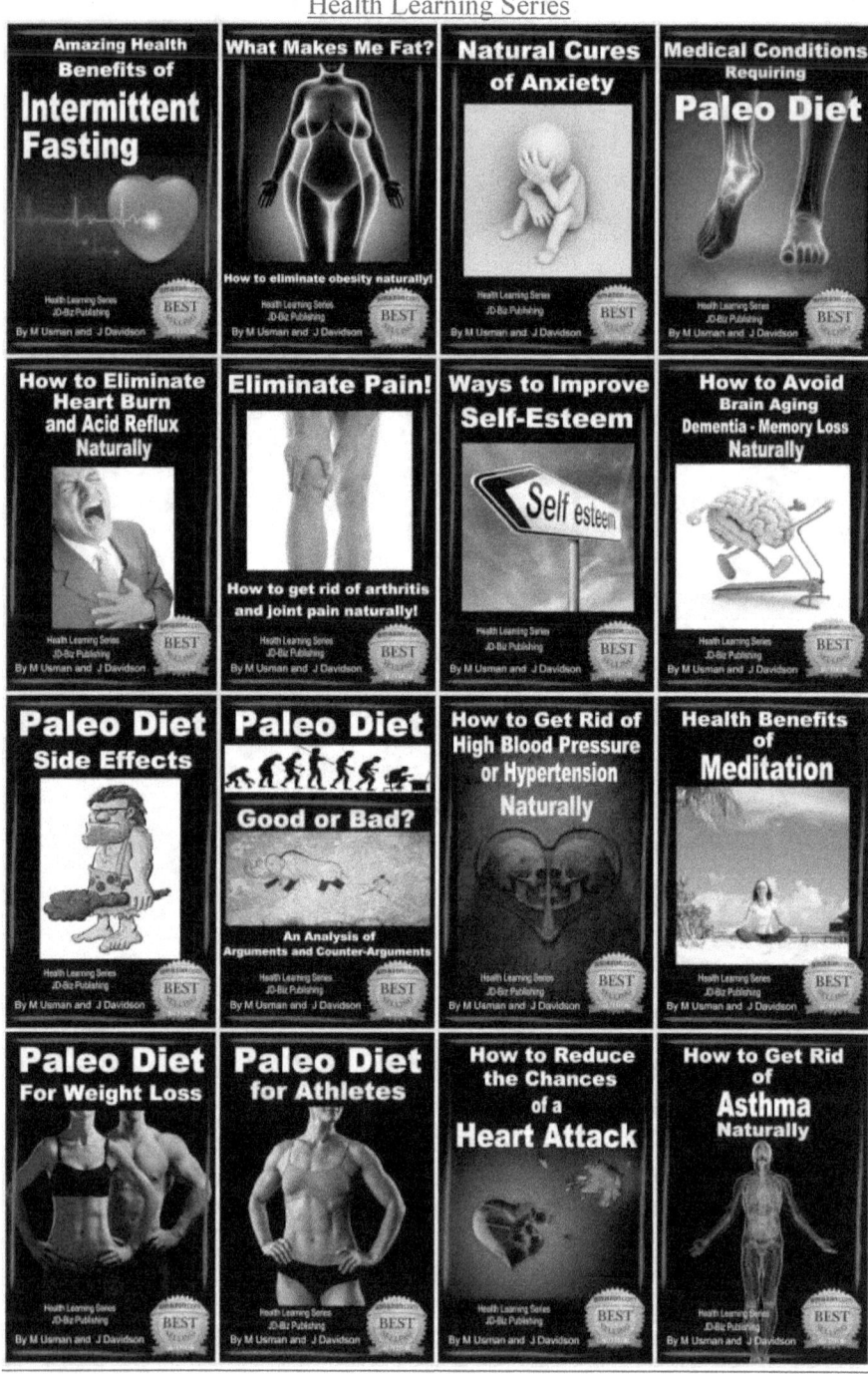

# Amazing Animal Book Series

Chinchillas · Beavers · Snakes · Dolphins · Wolves · Walruses

Polar Bears · Turtles · Bees · Frogs · Horses · Monkeys

Dinosaurs · Sharks · Whales · Spiders · Big Cats · Big Mammals of Yellowstone

Animals of Australia · Sasquatch - Yeti Abominable Snowman Bigfoot · Giant Panda Bears · Kittens · Komodo Dragons · Lady Bugs

Animals of North America · Meerkats · Birds of North America · Penguins · Hamsters · Elephants

# Learn To Draw Series

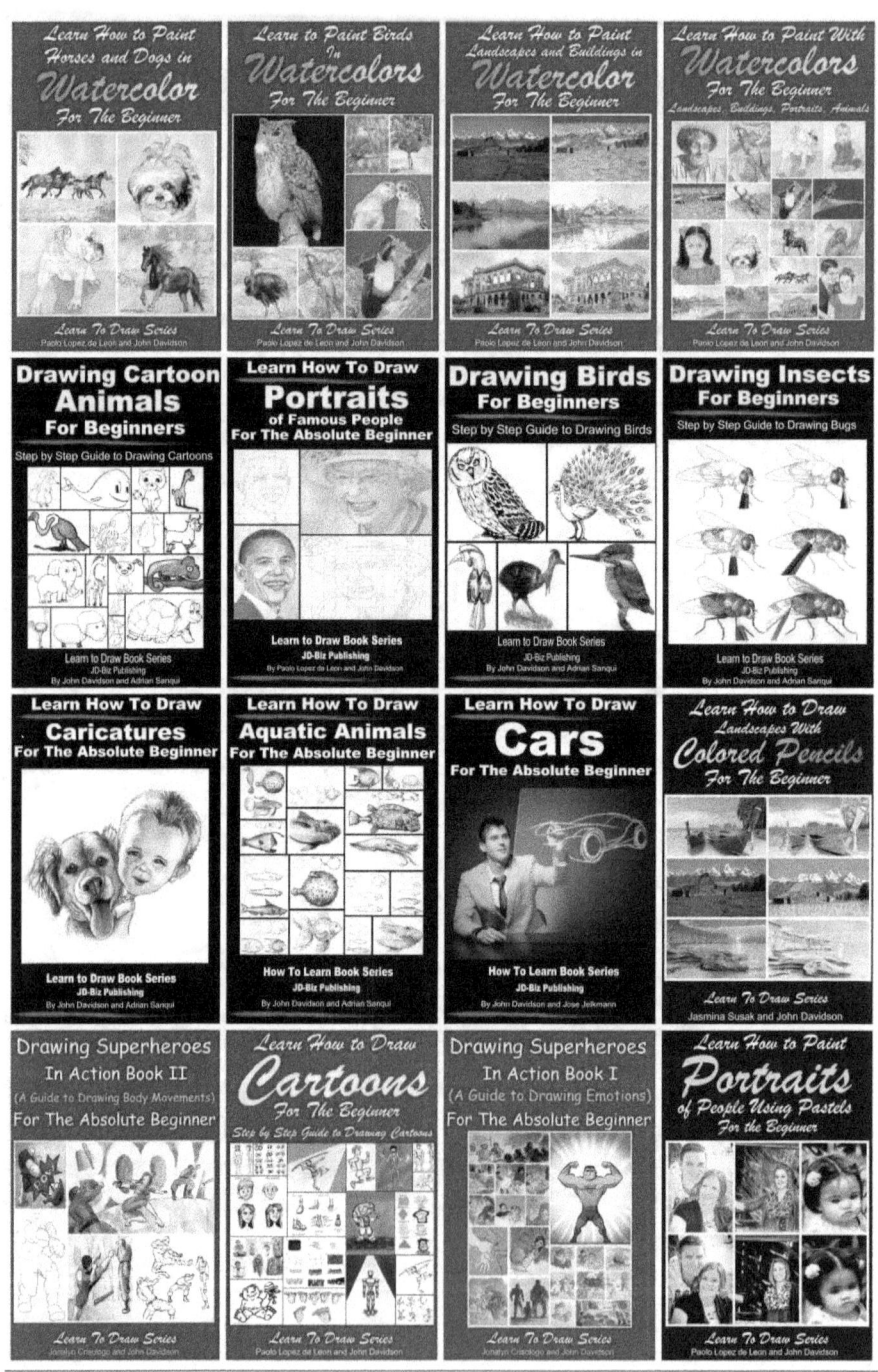

# How to Build and Plan Books

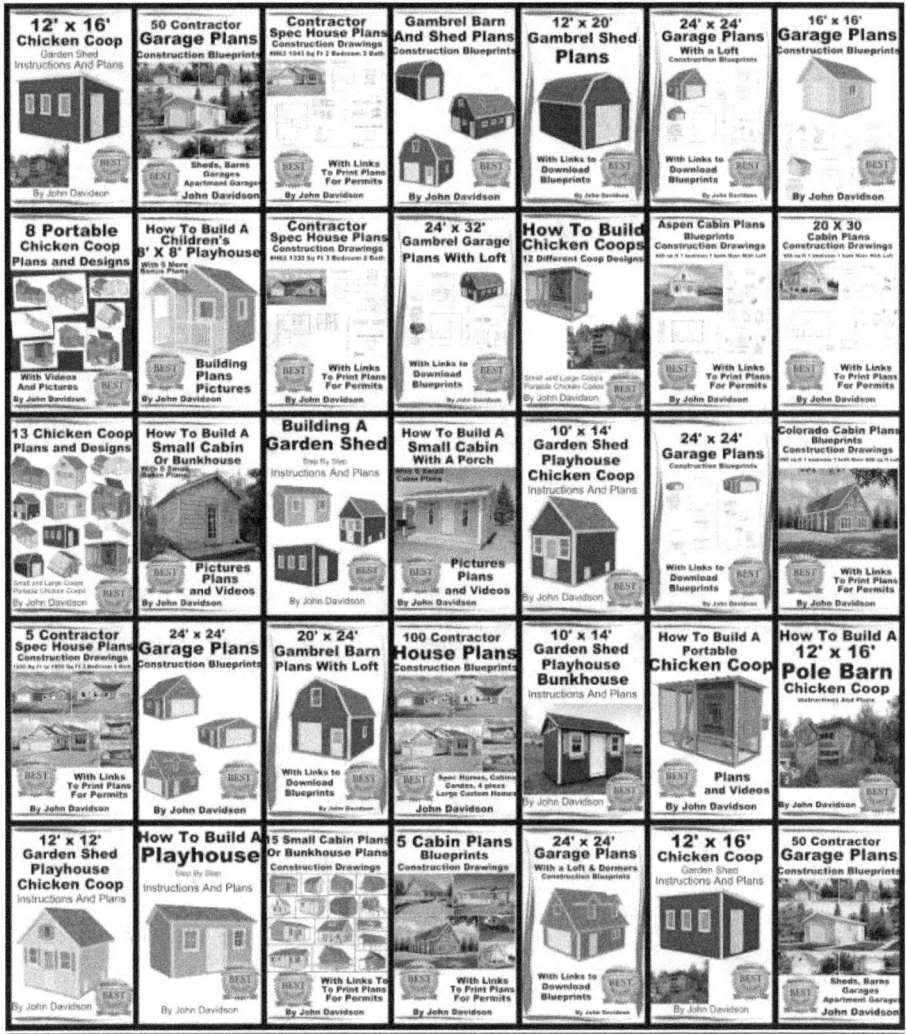

# Entrepreneur Book Series

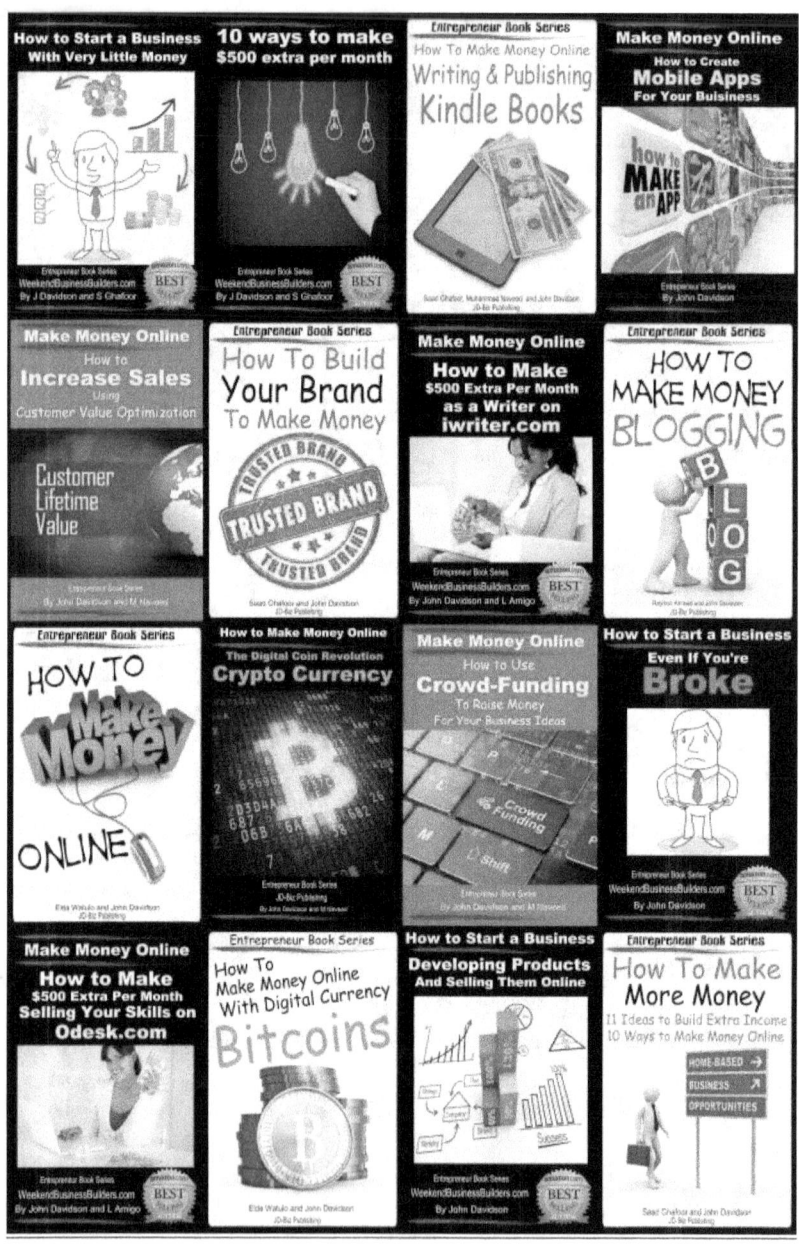

Our books are available at

1. Amazon.com

2. Barnes and Noble

3. Itunes

4. Kobo

5. Smashwords

6. Google Play Books

# Publisher

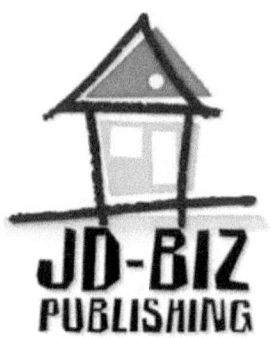

JD-Biz Corp

P O Box 374

Mendon, Utah 84325

http://www.jd-biz.com/

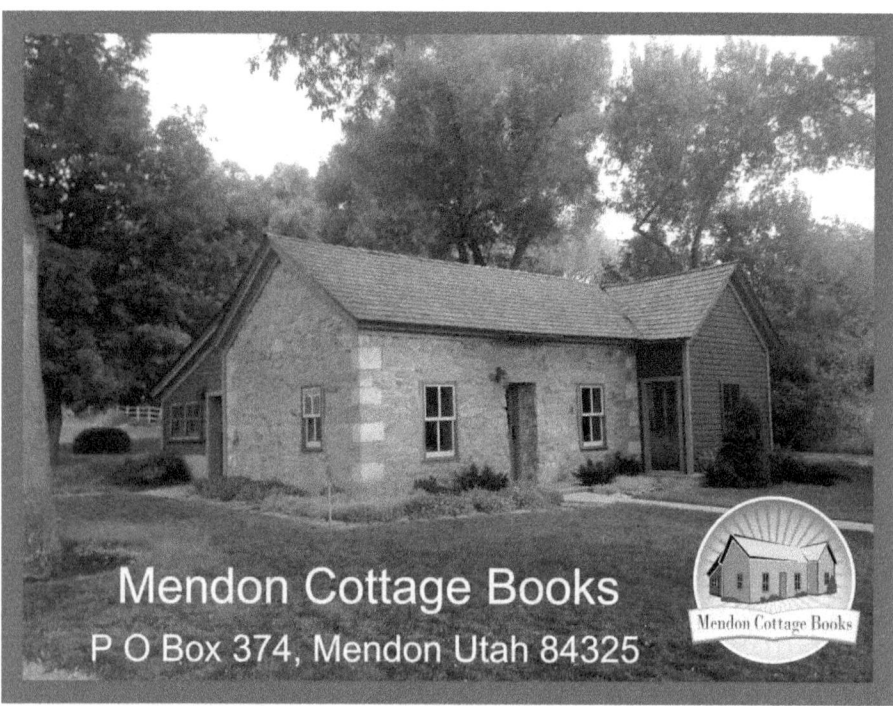

www.ingramcontent.com/pod-product-compliance
Lightning Source LLC
Chambersburg PA
CBHW071142280526
45787CB00003B/1380